Collagen Diet

A Women's 3-Week Step-by-Step Guide for Smoother Skin and Weight Loss with Recipes and a Meal Plan

copyright © 2023 Stephanie Hinderock

All rights reserved No part of this book may be reproduced, or stored in a retrieval system, or transmitted in any form or by any means, electronic, mechanical, photocopying, recording, or otherwise, without express written permission of the publisher.

Disclaimer

By reading this disclaimer, you are accepting the terms of the disclaimer in full. If you disagree with this disclaimer, please do not read the guide.

All of the content within this guide is provided for informational and educational purposes only, and should not be accepted as independent medical or other professional advice. The author is not a doctor, physician, nurse, mental health provider, or registered nutritionist/dietician. Therefore, using and reading this guide does not establish any form of a physician-patient relationship.

Always consult with a physician or another qualified health provider with any issues or questions you might have regarding any sort of medical condition. Do not ever disregard any qualified professional medical advice or delay seeking that advice because of anything you have read in this guide. The information in this guide is not intended to be any sort of medical advice and should not be used in lieu of any medical advice by a licensed and qualified medical professional.

The information in this guide has been compiled from a variety of known sources. However, the author cannot attest to or guarantee the accuracy of each source and thus should not be held liable for any errors or omissions.

You acknowledge that the publisher of this guide will not be held liable for any loss or damage of any kind incurred as a result of this guide or the reliance on any information provided within this guide. You acknowledge and agree that you assume all risk and responsibility for any action you undertake in response to the information in this guide.

Using this guide does not guarantee any particular result (e.g., weight loss or a cure). By reading this guide, you acknowledge that there are no guarantees to any specific outcome or results you can expect.

All product names, diet plans, or names used in this guide are for identification purposes only and are the property of their respective owners. The use of these names does not imply endorsement. All other trademarks cited herein are the property of their respective owners.

Where applicable, this guide is not intended to be a substitute for the original work of this diet plan and is, at most, a supplement to the original work for this diet plan and never a direct substitute. This guide is a personal expression of the facts of that diet plan.

Where applicable, persons shown in the cover images are stock photography models and the publisher has obtained the rights to use the images through license agreements with third-party stock image companies.

Table of Contents

Introduction 7
What Is Collagen? 10
    Common Types of Collagen 10
    Functions of Collagen 11
    Health Benefits of Collagen 12
    How Does Collagen Function in Our Body? 14
Collagen-Rich Foods 18
    Animal-Based Sources of Collagen 18
    Plant-Based Boosters for Collagen Production 19
    Highlighting the Importance of Variety in Your Diet 20
The Multifaceted Benefits of Collagen for Women 21
    Combating Cellulite 21
    Assisting in Weight Management 22
    Supporting Pregnancy and Postpartum Recovery 23
    Backed by Ongoing Research 24
The Collagen Diet 25
    Principles of the Collagen Diet 25
    Other Benefits of the Collagen Diet 27
    Disadvantages of The Collagen Diet 29
3-Week Collagen Diet Plan 31
    Incorporating Collagen into Your Diet 31
    Addressing Common Misconceptions 31
    The Modern Diet and Collagen 32
    Week 1 – Mental Preparation for a Collagen-Rich Diet 32
    Week 2 – Curating Your Collagen-Rich Food and Recipe List 35
    Week 3 – Crafting Your Weekly Collagen-Rich Diet Plan 37
    Foods to Eat in a Collagen Diet 40
    Foods to Avoid in a Collagen Diet 41

One-Week Sample Plan	**43**
Sample Recipes for Collagen Diet	**46**
Avocado Deviled Eggs	47
Braised Beef with Garlic and Thyme	49
Raw Kale Salad	51
Bone Broth	53
Seared Salmon	55
Steamed Salmon	57
New York Strip Steak	59
Lettuce-Wrapped Bison Burger	61
Veggie and Egg Frittata	63
Spinach Salad	65
Turkey Meatballs	67
Conclusion	**69**
FAQ	**72**
References and Helpful Links	**75**

Introduction

In recent years, the collagen diet has emerged as a popular choice for individuals seeking to improve their overall health and wellness. This diet centers around consuming foods high in collagen, a protein vital for maintaining the body's structural integrity. The aim is to support skin health, joint flexibility, and general vitality.

Have you heard about the collagen diet? It's not just another trend sweeping through the wellness community. With a foundation in nutrition science, this approach focuses on boosting collagen intake—a key protein that plays a crucial role in our bodies. From keeping our skin supple to ensuring our joints move smoothly, collagen's importance cannot be overstated.

The diet itself isn't complicated. It involves incorporating specific foods into your meals that are rich in collagen or promote collagen production within the body. Think of bone broth, chicken, fish, leafy greens, berries, and garlic, to name a few. These aren't just good for you; they're also delicious and versatile, making it easy to stick with the plan. Besides the dietary aspect, the collagen diet often includes lifestyle recommendations, such as staying hydrated and avoiding excessive sugar intake, which can degrade collagen levels.

But why consider the collagen diet? For starters, it's about more than just looking good. It's about feeling strong, flexible, and vibrant at any age. Users of the collagen diet report experiencing smoother skin, fewer joint pains, and a general sense of well-being. These aren't baseless claims; they're backed by an understanding of how collagen works in the body and the effects of boosting its levels through diet.

In this guide, we will talk about the following;

- What is Collagen?
- Common Types, Functions of Collagen
- How Collagen Works in Our Body
- Health Benefits of Collagen
- Collagen Diet
- Collagen-Rich Foods
- 3-Week Collagen Diet Plan
- Sample Meal Plan and Recipes

Embarking on the collagen diet doesn't require drastic changes. It's about making mindful choices, adding nutrient-rich foods to your meals, and giving your body the building blocks it needs to thrive. Whether you're curious about how to get started or looking for ways to maintain a collagen-rich diet, this guide will provide you with the information you need to make informed decisions about your health and wellness.

By taking a closer look at the collagen diet, you'll discover how integrating collagen-rich foods and supportive lifestyle habits can contribute to your overall health goals. This guide aims to demystify the process, offering practical advice and insights to help you on your wellness journey.

What Is Collagen?

Collagen is the most abundant protein in the human body and plays a crucial role in providing structure and support to various tissues. It's a vital component of skin, bones, muscles, tendons, ligaments, blood vessels, and digestive systems. Collagen acts as a "glue" that helps hold the body together, maintaining strength, elasticity, and regeneration of tissues.

Common Types of Collagen

There are at least 16 types of collagen, but four main types are particularly important:

1. *Type I*: This variety comprises 90% of the collagen in your body and consists of tightly packed fibers. It plays a key role in maintaining the health of teeth, skin, bones, tendons, fibrous cartilage, and connective tissues.
2. *Type II*: Composed of fibers that are more loosely arranged, present in elastic cartilage that provides cushioning for your joints.
3. *Type III*: Supports the structure of muscles, organs, and arteries.

4. ***Type IV***: Helps with filtration and is found in the layers of your skin.

Each type of collagen supports the body in different ways and is critical to specific functions.

Functions of Collagen

The primary functions of collagen include:

- ***Structural Support***: Collagen fibers provide strength and structure to tissues throughout the body. In the skin, collagen contributes to firmness and suppleness. In bones, it acts as a scaffold that provides strength and flexibility.
- ***Skin Elasticity***: The resilience and elasticity of skin are attributed to collagen, which helps in the rapid turnover of skin cells and promotes youthful, healthy-looking skin.
- ***Joint and Bone Health***: Collagen is crucial for maintaining joint health by ensuring the integrity of cartilage, which protects joints. Its presence in bones also helps them to be strong yet flexible enough to absorb impact.
- ***Wound Healing***: Collagen plays a key role in wound healing by forming new fibrous tissue and helping in the repair process.
- ***Blood Vessel Function***: Type IV collagen, in particular, contributes to the formation of endothelial

cells that line blood vessels, supporting vascular health and function.

The body naturally produces collagen, but as we age, this production decreases, leading to common signs of aging such as wrinkles, sagging skin, and weaker joints and bones. This decline in collagen levels is one reason why dietary intake through collagen-rich foods or supplements has gained popularity for those looking to mitigate the effects of aging and support overall health.

Environmental factors such as smoking, high sugar consumption, and excessive sun exposure can also degrade collagen fibers, further emphasizing the importance of a healthy lifestyle and diet to maintain collagen levels.

Health Benefits of Collagen

When it comes to health benefits, collagen offers much more than just keeping skin looking youthful. Some of the potential benefits of incorporating collagen into your diet or skincare routine include:

Skin Health

Collagen plays a crucial role in maintaining the youthful appearance and elasticity of the skin. It helps to reduce wrinkles, improve skin hydration, and promote a vibrant, healthy glow. By providing structural support, it enhances the skin's overall texture and firmness.

As collagen levels decline with age, supplementing with or increasing dietary intake of collagen can help counteract the effects of aging, leading to smoother, more supple skin.

Joint Health

The integrity and functionality of joints are significantly supported by collagen. It contributes to the strength and flexibility of cartilage, the tissue that protects joints. Adequate collagen levels can help reduce the risk of joint degeneration and the symptoms of disorders such as osteoarthritis.

Many people report a decrease in joint pain and improved mobility after incorporating collagen supplements into their diet, highlighting its importance in maintaining joint health.

Bone Strength

Collagen is a major component of bones, contributing to their structure and strength. It works synergistically with calcium and other minerals to ensure bone density and resilience. With aging, diminished collagen production can lead to weaker bones and conditions like osteoporosis. Supplementing with collagen has been shown to support bone health by enhancing bone mineral density and offering protection against bone loss.

Gut Health

Emerging research suggests that collagen may have beneficial effects on gut health. Its amino acid composition, particularly glycine and proline, supports the repair and integrity of the intestinal lining. This can contribute to a healthier gut barrier, potentially preventing issues like leaky gut syndrome, which has been linked to various autoimmune diseases and chronic health conditions. Collagen's anti-inflammatory properties also play a role in promoting a healthy digestive system.

In summary, collagen's contribution to the body extends far beyond its structural duties. Its impact on skin health, joint health, bone strength, and gut health underscores its importance in overall well-being and the prevention of age-related decline. Incorporating collagen-rich foods or supplements into one's diet can be a valuable strategy for enhancing personal health and vitality.

How Does Collagen Function in Our Body?

Collagen functions in our body through several mechanisms, primarily by providing structural support and promoting the health and integrity of tissues. Here's a detailed look at how collagen works across different aspects of our body:

1. **Structural Support and Tissue Repair**
   - *Skin*: Collagen is a major component of the skin, accounting for about 75-80% of its dry weight. It provides the skin with structure, elasticity, and

resilience. By doing so, collagen helps in the process of skin renewal and healing, contributing to a youthful appearance.

- **Bones and Joints**: In bones, collagen works alongside calcium and other minerals to provide strength and flexibility. It forms a scaffold that supports the bone's mineral content. In joints, collagen is a vital part of cartilage, the rubber-like tissue that protects the ends of bones from friction. Adequate collagen keeps cartilage strong and prevents it from deteriorating, which is crucial for joint function and mobility.
- **Tendons and Ligaments**: These are composed mainly of collagen. Tendons connect muscles to bones, while ligaments connect bones to each other. Collagen gives these tissues the strength and elasticity needed to absorb impact and facilitate movement.

2. **Wound Healing**

Collagen plays a critical role in wound healing by forming new fibrous tissue that replaces damaged skin. It acts as a protective barrier for new tissue growth and provides a platform for the growth of new cells. This process is essential not only for skin injuries but also for internal wounds.

3. **Gut Health**

Though research is still evolving, collagen is believed to contribute to gut health by supporting the lining of the gastrointestinal tract. Its amino acids may help maintain the integrity of the gut wall, potentially preventing issues like leaky gut syndrome, where toxins and bacteria enter the bloodstream through gaps in the intestinal walls.

4. Blood Vessel and Heart Health

Collagen contributes to the structure and flexibility of blood vessels. Type IV collagen, in particular, forms part of the basal lamina layer of the endothelium (the inner lining of blood vessels), supporting vascular integrity and function. A healthy vascular system is essential for heart health and efficient circulation throughout the body.

Mechanism of Action

On a molecular level, collagen's structure is characterized by long, stiff, triple-stranded helices. These helices pack together to form fibrils, which in turn create the fibers that provide tensile strength and structure to tissues. In the body, collagen is continuously being broken down and replaced.

This dynamic process requires a supply of amino acids (particularly proline, glycine, and hydroxyproline), vitamin C, zinc, and copper—nutrients that either contribute directly to the synthesis of collagen or act as cofactors in enzymatic processes that stabilize the collagen helix and promote cross-linking between collagen molecules.

Understanding how collagen works underscores its importance in maintaining overall health, highlighting why dietary intake and supplementation can be beneficial, especially as natural production declines with age.

Collagen-Rich Foods

Incorporating collagen-rich foods into your diet is a holistic approach to boosting collagen levels in the body, which in turn supports skin health, joint flexibility, bone strength, and gut health. While the body naturally produces collagen, aging, and environmental factors can slow down its production. Thus, consuming foods high in collagen or that support its production is beneficial.

Here's a breakdown of both animal-based sources of collagen and plant-based foods that promote collagen production:

Animal-Based Sources of Collagen

- *Bone Broth*: Made by simmering bones and connective tissue, bone broth is a rich source of collagen. It also contains other nutrients that support joint and gut health.
- *Fish and Shellfish*: The skin of fish and shellfish is packed with collagen. Marine collagen is especially easy for the body to absorb and utilize.

- **Chicken Skin**: Chicken skin is another excellent source of collagen, particularly Type I collagen, which benefits the skin and tendons.
- **Pork and Beef Cuts**: Cuts of meat that contain more connective tissue, such as brisket, ribs, and shank, are higher in collagen. Slow cooking these cuts can help in extracting collagen.

Plant-Based Boosters for Collagen Production

Although plants do not contain collagen, certain foods can support collagen production in the body through their nutrient content:

- *Garlic*: It contains sulfur, a necessary component for collagen synthesis in the body. Garlic also has taurine and lipid acid, which help rebuild damaged collagen fibers.
- *Berries*: Rich in antioxidants, berries such as strawberries, blueberries, and raspberries can protect collagen in the skin from damage.
- *Soy Products*: Soy contains genistein, an isoflavone that blocks enzymes detrimental to collagen while promoting collagen production. Tofu, tempeh, and soy milk are good sources.
- *Citrus Fruits*: Vitamin C-rich fruits like oranges, lemons, and grapefruits play a critical role in collagen

synthesis. Vitamin C acts as a co-factor in proline and lysine hydroxylation, a necessary step in collagen formation.

Highlighting the Importance of Variety in Your Diet

A diversified diet ensures a broad spectrum of nutrients essential for collagen production and overall health. For non-vegetarians, incorporating animal-based collagen sources can directly supply the body with collagen. Vegetarians and vegans, on the other hand, can focus on plant-based foods that enhance collagen production. Both approaches are valid and can be tailored according to dietary preferences and restrictions.

Balancing your intake of collagen-rich foods with those that promote its production helps maintain optimal levels of this crucial protein. Hence, integrating a variety of these foods into your daily diet can contribute significantly to your physical well-being and anti-aging efforts.

The Multifaceted Benefits of Collagen for Women

Women derive numerous benefits from collagen, a versatile protein that addresses several female-specific health concerns.

Combating Cellulite

Contrary to the common misconception, cellulite primarily affects women more than men. This condition, which presents as lumpy and dimpled flesh primarily on the thighs, buttocks, or hips, is the result of fats and dead cells accumulating beneath the skin's surface. It's important to understand that cellulite's formation is influenced by factors such as hormones, genetics, diet, and lifestyle choices.

Collagen, a crucial protein in our bodies, plays a significant role in addressing this issue. It works to repair and strengthen the fibers that connect the skin to the underlying flesh. By doing so, collagen can significantly smooth out the appearance of cellulite and firm up the skin in these affected areas, offering a more toned and even appearance. This insight into the causes and solutions for cellulite sheds light on the importance of a healthy lifestyle and proper skin care regimen in maintaining smooth, firm skin.

Assisting in Weight Management

Collagen is increasingly recognized for its role in supporting weight loss efforts, primarily through its effective suppression of appetite. Studies have shown that collagen is approximately 40% more satiating than other commonly consumed proteins such as whey, soy, and casein. This higher satiety level is crucial for those looking to reduce their overall calorie intake without feeling deprived.

Further research into collagen's effects on the body reveals that it can enhance the release of satiety hormones. These hormones play a pivotal role in signaling to our brains that we are full, thus leading to a significant reduction in the urge to consume more food. This mechanism has been linked to a notable 20% decrease in food consumption at meals following the intake of collagen.

This evidence suggests that incorporating collagen supplements into one's diet could be a strategic addition to a comprehensive weight management plan, providing a natural and effective means to control appetite and reduce overall calorie intake.

Supporting Pregnancy and Postpartum Recovery

During and after pregnancy, many women experience a range of physical changes, some of the most noticeable being alterations in hair and skin condition. Specifically, it's common to observe hair becoming dry and brittle, losing its natural luster and strength. Similarly, the skin may lose some of its elasticity, resulting in a less firm appearance. This is where the benefits of collagen supplementation come into play.

Incorporating collagen into one's diet can significantly revitalize hair health, effectively restoring its shine and strength to levels often seen before pregnancy. This means that hair not only looks better but is also healthier and more resilient. Beyond hair, collagen plays a critical role in enhancing skin elasticity. This is particularly beneficial when it comes to tightening sagging abdominal skin that many women experience following childbirth.

Moreover, collagen's impact extends beyond mere aesthetic improvements. Its role during this critical period of a woman's life highlights its adaptability to meet unique nutritional needs, thereby promoting overall health and wellness. By supporting skin and hair health, collagen supplementation can also contribute to a woman's emotional well-being and self-confidence post-pregnancy, making it a valuable addition to postpartum care routines.

Backed by Ongoing Research

The effectiveness of collagen in enhancing women's health is supported by research across various skin types. Studies with female participants have revealed positive subjective assessments, with many reporting notable improvements in skin appearance.

Additionally, these studies confirmed that collagen use was free of side effects and well-tolerated throughout the research. Ongoing scientific inquiries continue to unveil the nutritional dynamics and processes through which collagen supplementation fosters better skin physiology and aesthetics.

The evidence underscores collagen's broad spectrum of benefits for women, addressing issues from cellulite and weight management to pregnancy-related changes and skin health. With its wide-ranging positive effects on the body and well-being, collagen emerges as a crucial nutrient for women's health optimization.

The Collagen Diet

When it comes to incorporating collagen into one's diet, there are several options available. Some people choose to take supplements, which can come in various forms such as pills, powders, or even gummies. Others prefer to consume collagen-rich foods like bone broth, fish, and lean meats.

One popular trend in recent years is the "collagen diet," where individuals follow a specific meal plan focused on incorporating collagen-rich foods into their daily diet. This approach is believed to provide a more natural and holistic way of increasing collagen levels in the body.

Principles of the Collagen Diet

The principles of the collagen diet revolve around optimizing your body's collagen production and preservation to support skin health, joint health, and overall well-being. Here's a concise overview of its core tenets:

1. *Increase Collagen Intake*: Focus on consuming foods and supplements that are rich in collagen, such as bone broth, chicken, fish, egg whites, and specific collagen

supplements. The goal is to directly boost your body's collagen levels.

2. ***Support Collagen Production***: Prioritize foods high in nutrients that aid collagen synthesis. Vitamin C from citrus fruits, leafy greens, and berries, zinc from nuts and seeds, and copper found in shellfish are essential for collagen production.

3. ***Protect Existing Collagen***: Incorporate antioxidants into your diet through fruits, vegetables, and other whole foods to protect your body's collagen from oxidative damage. Foods rich in vitamins A and E, like carrots, sweet potatoes, and almonds, can help shield collagen fibers.

4. ***Limit Collagen Damage***: Avoid or minimize intake of sugar, refined carbs, excessive alcohol, and processed foods, as these can interfere with collagen repair and accelerate its breakdown. Such dietary habits contribute to inflammation and advanced glycation end products (AGEs), which negatively impact collagen.

5. ***Stay Hydrated***: Water is crucial for maintaining the integrity of the skin's collagen structure. Proper hydration ensures that collagen fibers remain supple and less prone to damage.

6. ***Healthy Lifestyle Choices***: Beyond diet, engaging in regular exercise, protecting your skin from excessive sun exposure, and avoiding smoking can further enhance collagen production and preservation. These

lifestyle choices complement your diet in supporting overall collagen health.

7. ***Holistic Nutritional Approach***: Rather than focusing solely on collagen, ensure your diet is balanced and rich in a variety of nutrients. A holistic approach supports not only collagen health but also overall physical wellness.

By adhering to these principles, the collagen diet aims to improve skin elasticity, reduce wrinkles, strengthen joints, and promote a radiant and youthful appearance through natural and dietary means.

Other Benefits of the Collagen Diet

Apart from the well-known benefits for skin elasticity, joint health, and bone strength, the collagen diet offers several other advantages that contribute to overall wellness and bodily function. Here are some additional benefits:

1. ***Boosted Muscle Mass***: Collagen is a protein that plays a crucial role in maintaining muscle tissue. A collagen-rich diet can support muscle growth and repair, which is especially beneficial for individuals engaged in regular physical activity or those looking to increase their muscle mass.
2. ***Hair and Nail Strength***: Just like it benefits the skin, collagen can also enhance the strength and appearance

of hair and nails by providing the protein building blocks needed for growth and preventing brittleness.
3. ***Improved Sleep Quality***: Glycine, an amino acid abundant in collagen, has been shown to improve sleep quality. It can help in falling asleep more quickly, reducing symptoms of insomnia, and promoting a deeper, more restful night's sleep.
4. ***Enhanced Brain Health***: Preliminary research suggests that collagen consumption could have protective effects on brain health, including potential benefits for mood and reducing anxiety levels. Glycine, in particular, plays a role in the central nervous system and neurotransmitter functions.
5. ***Supports Liver Health***: Glycine also helps in detoxifying the body by supporting liver function in processing and eliminating toxins. A collagen-rich diet may contribute to improved liver health and detoxification pathways.

By incorporating collagen-rich foods and supplements into your diet, you're not just investing in your appearance but bolstering your body's overall health and functionality. These diverse benefits underscore the importance of collagen not only as a cosmetic enhancer but also as a crucial component of a holistic approach to wellness.

Disadvantages of The Collagen Diet

While the collagen diet comes with a host of health benefits, it's important to recognize there may be some disadvantages or considerations to keep in mind. However, it's widely understood that the benefits often outweigh these potential downsides:

1. *Allergies and Sensitivities*: Individuals with allergies to common sources of collagen, such as fish, shellfish, or eggs, might find it challenging to follow a collagen diet without experiencing adverse reactions. Careful selection of collagen sources is necessary to avoid allergens.
2. *Dietary Restrictions*: Those who adhere to vegetarian or vegan diets may find it difficult to incorporate traditional sources of collagen, which are primarily animal-based. Though there are plant-based alternatives that support collagen production, direct collagen sources are animal-derived.
3. *Cost Considerations*: High-quality collagen supplements and collagen-rich foods can be more expensive than other nutrients or protein sources. This might make the collagen diet an investment for some, potentially limiting its accessibility.
4. *Limited Research in Some Areas*: While the benefits of collagen for skin health, joint health, and bone density are supported by research, other purported

benefits of the collagen diet might have less scientific backing, requiring individuals to manage their expectations.

5. ***Overemphasis on One Nutrient***: Focusing too intently on collagen could lead some individuals to neglect the importance of a balanced diet rich in a variety of nutrients necessary for overall health.

Despite these potential drawbacks, the use of collagen in various forms has gained popularity in recent years. Research continues to explore the efficacy and safety of collagen supplements and diets, with promising results.

3-Week Collagen Diet Plan

Before devising a comprehensive dietary plan, it's essential to understand the significance of collagen and its various types. Here is a structured approach to considering collagen in your diet:

Incorporating Collagen into Your Diet

- *Multi-Collagen Products*: To ensure a well-rounded intake, consider multi-collagen products. These can help you achieve a balanced consumption of the different collagen types.
- *Daily Servings*: For optimal benefit, include 1 to 3 servings of collagen in your daily diet. This recommendation is particularly crucial from age 25 onwards when natural collagen production begins to wane.

Addressing Common Misconceptions

Some may question the efficacy of dietary collagen, believing it doesn't translate directly into bodily collagen in joints, ligaments, and the gut. However, the process is more nuanced:

- ***Collagen Digestion***: Consumed collagen is hydrolyzed in the stomach, breaking down into amino acids such as proline, hydroxyproline, and glycine. These amino acids then act as the foundational building blocks for the body's collagen production, facilitating a natural synthesis rather than an immediate "transplant."

The Modern Diet and Collagen

Today's diets often lack the rich collagen sources found in traditional diets, such as stocks, soups, and bone broths. This change contributes to a decrease in both collagen consumption and production, impacting our external appearance and internal structure. By incorporating collagen-rich foods or supplements, we can counteract these effects, supporting both beauty and bodily function.

Following is a diet plan sample and preparations to do:

Week 1 – Mental Preparation for a Collagen-Rich Diet

The Importance of Mental Readiness

Starting any new diet requires a significant mental shift. It's not merely about changing what you eat; it's about transforming how you think about food. This week is dedicated to mentally preparing yourself for the major lifestyle adjustment ahead. Remember, mental readiness is the bedrock of successful dietary changes.

Commitment: The Initial Step

The initial two days should focus on commitment. During this period, repeat to yourself the importance of incorporating collagen into your diet. This mantra-like repetition, "collagen, collagen, collagen," serves as a mental cue, reinforcing your decision until you feel fully prepared to start this new chapter.

Clearing the Dietary Clutter

The following couple of days will involve identifying and deciding to eliminate foods that hinder your goals. Favorites though they might be, items such as soda, popcorn, mayonnaise, white bread, salty snacks, processed, sugary, and fried foods must be recognized for their counterproductive effects on your health and diet. It's time to firmly say goodbye to these culprits, clearing the way for more nutritious choices.

Welcoming Supportive Foods

Once you've made space by eliminating unhelpful foods, the next step is to introduce and celebrate foods that align with your new collagen-boosting diet. This isn't just about restriction; it's also about discovery and enjoyment.

Identify foods that not only delight your palate but also support specific health targets, whether that's heart health, tendon and cartilage strengthening, fat reduction, or skin rejuvenation. Given the multifaceted benefits of many foods, prioritize those with targeted benefits to meet your specific health objectives.

Planning with Flexibility and Realism

While planning, adopt a flexible and realistic approach. Recognize that completely overhauling your diet won't be straightforward. There will be challenges and occasional slip-ups. It's important to mentally prepare for these moments, accepting them without harsh self-judgment. Understand that mistakes are part of the human experience; what matters is your response and commitment to not repeating them.

Accepting Mistakes and Moving Forward

Prepare yourself mentally for potential setbacks. Whether it's succumbing to a craving or accidentally deviating from your diet plan, it's vital to approach such instances with kindness and understanding towards yourself. Acknowledge these moments, learn from them, and then continue forward with renewed determination.

The Culinary Adventure Begins

Having spent seven days getting mentally prepared, you're now ready for the practical aspects of your collagen-rich diet. The next step involves creating a detailed list of recipes and the necessary ingredients. This list isn't just a shopping guide—it's the foundation of your culinary adventures, offering a tangible way to bring your diet plan to life.

This initial week is crucial for setting a positive tone for your dietary changes. By focusing on mental readiness, commitment, and planning, you're laying the groundwork for a successful transition to a healthier, collagen-rich lifestyle.

Week 2 – Curating Your Collagen-Rich Food and Recipe List

Unveiling the Transition Phase

The second week marks a crucial period in your dietary overhaul, which we might aptly term the "Transition Phase" or, alternatively, the "Practice Phase." This timeframe is dedicated to gradually acquainting your body with a new nutritional regimen centered around collagen.

It's about weaving one collagen-infused recipe into your daily meals, gradually expanding your dietary palette without overwhelming yourself or your digestive system.

Experimentation and Introduction of New Foods

Imagine starting your day with a nourishing smoothie crafted from gelatin, mixed berries, spirulina, and almond milk, or revitalizing your lunchtime routine with a hearty chicken soup enriched with bone broth.

These meals serve as your initial foray into the world of collagen-rich dining. Document each recipe, paying close attention to the ingredients, as they'll become your toolkit for future culinary creations.

Day-by-Day Diversification

Progressing through the week, introduce variety by incorporating different collagen-rich foods into your meals, such as pumpkin seeds or hard-boiled eggs. This methodical integration allows you to explore new tastes and textures while ensuring you're not overloading your plate with too many options at once. As you make these adjustments, naturally, some of the less beneficial food items will fall by the wayside, making room for more nutrient-dense choices.

Gradual Reduction and Replacement

This approach offers the dual benefit of introducing new, beneficial foods into your diet while simultaneously reducing reliance on less nutritious options.

Each new collagen-rich addition to your diet should be noted, building a comprehensive list that supports a wide range of meal combinations and ensures you never find yourself stuck in a dietary rut.

Extending the Transition

Recognize that the transition phase is flexible; it can be extended beyond Week 2 into Weeks 3 and 4 if you find the pace more comfortable or if you're still exploring collagen-rich food options. This extended "get-to-know-you" period with new foods allows for a smoother, more sustainable shift towards a diet that consistently incorporates the recommended daily servings of 1-3 collagen-packed meals.

Moving Towards a Collagen-Forward Diet

By the end of this phase, the goal is to have seamlessly integrated collagen-rich foods into your daily routine, setting the stage for the final transition where your diet is rich in collagen, meeting your body's needs for this vital protein.

This thoughtful, phased approach ensures that your move to a collagen-centric diet is not only manageable but enjoyable, paving the way for lasting health benefits and a deeper appreciation of nourishing, wholesome foods.

Week 3 – Crafting Your Weekly Collagen-Rich Diet Plan

Elevating Breakfast with Nutrient-Packed Choices

As you enter Week 3, it's time to solidify your commitment to a collagen-rich diet by outlining a detailed weekly meal plan. Begin your mornings with a diverse array of energizing breakfast options designed to kickstart your day.

Consider integrating smoothies blended with a mix of fruits and vegetables, eggs prepared in various styles for protein, turmeric tea for its anti-inflammatory benefits, and a side of spinach, berries, mushrooms, or potatoes. These choices not only offer a delicious start to the day but also contribute to your collagen intake.

Diversifying Lunch with Healthy, Hearty Options

Lunch can be an exciting mix of flavors and nutrients. While salads packed with vibrant vegetables serve as a staple for many, introducing variety will keep your diet interesting and enjoyable.

Alternate between bone broth or chicken soup days to provide your body with the essential amino acids needed for collagen production. These light yet satisfying options will fuel your afternoons without weighing you down.

Delightful Dinners to Look Forward To

When it comes to dinner, focus on incorporating collagen-boosting foods that also comfort and satisfy. Options like steamed broccoli, accompanied by protein-rich turkey meatballs, guacamole for healthy fats, shredded salsa chicken for a flavorful twist, or simply grilled chicken, offer versatile and nutritious ways to end your day. Each of these dinners supports your body's collagen synthesis while providing a delightful culinary experience.

Snacking Smart with Collagen-Supportive Treats

Snacks are an integral part of maintaining energy levels throughout the day, and choosing collagen-friendly options is key. Greek yogurt, loaded with protein, serves as an excellent base for fruit or nuts.

Avocado Devilled eggs offer a twist on a classic, packing both flavor and nutritional benefits. Other great snack options include chicken breast paired with broccoli, steam-cooked vegetables for a light bite, or salsa chicken for a zesty treat. These snacks are not only delicious but also align with your goals of increasing collagen intake.

The Importance of a Well-Rounded Approach

This week is crucial for establishing a well-rounded collagen-rich diet that encompasses all meals and snacks. By carefully selecting ingredients and recipes that boost collagen production, you ensure that your body receives the nutrients it needs to support skin health, joint function, and overall well-being. This comprehensive approach lays the foundation for a sustainable dietary lifestyle that prioritizes health and enjoyment in equal measure.

In crafting your weekly plan, remember to consider variety, balance, and personal taste preferences to create a menu that's both beneficial and enjoyable. This detailed planning phase is instrumental in successfully integrating a collagen-rich diet into your life, setting you up for noticeable health improvements and a deeper appreciation for nutrient-dense foods.

Foods to Eat in a Collagen Diet

When focusing on a diet to boost collagen, aim to include:

1. **Bone Broth**: Rich in collagen, bone broth also offers various amino acids essential for collagen synthesis.
2. **Chicken**: A major source of collagen, chicken contains connective tissues that are packed with this protein.
3. **Fish and Shellfish**: Their bones and ligaments are great sources of collagen. Wild salmon, in particular, is beneficial for its high omega-3 content.
4. **Egg Whites**: Contain large amounts of proline, an amino acid important for collagen production.
5. **Berries**: Strawberries, blueberries, blackberries, and raspberries are rich in antioxidants that protect the skin's collagen.
6. **Citrus Fruits**: High in vitamin C, fruits like oranges, lemons, and limes help in collagen synthesis.
7. **Leafy Greens**: Vegetables such as spinach and kale are high in vitamin C and antioxidants, promoting collagen production and protection.
8. **Garlic**: It contains sulfur, which helps synthesize and prevent the breakdown of collagen.

9. ***Nuts and Seeds***: Almonds and sunflower seeds are packed with vitamin E, an antioxidant that can help protect collagen in the skin.
10. Tomatoes: Another excellent source of vitamin C and also contains lycopene, an antioxidant that supports skin health.

Foods to Avoid in a Collagen Diet

To protect your body's collagen, consider reducing or eliminating:

1. ***Sugary Treats and Beverages***: Sugar can interfere with collagen's ability to repair itself.
2. ***Processed Meats***: High in sulfites and other preservatives that can weaken collagen production.
3. ***White Bread and Pastas***: Refined carbs can lead to inflammation, indirectly breaking down collagen.
4. ***Fried Foods***: High in trans fats that can contribute to oxidative stress, damaging collagen and elastin in the skin.
5. ***Alcohol***: Excessive consumption can lead to dehydration, affecting the skin's collagen levels.
6. ***Caffeinated Beverages***: In large quantities, caffeine can reduce collagen production, but moderation is key as it can be part of a balanced diet.

By focusing on nutrient-rich foods that support collagen production and avoiding those that can harm it, you can effectively contribute to your overall skin health and wellness through your diet.

One-Week Sample Plan

We know it can be overwhelming to completely revamp your diet, so here is a sample plan for incorporating collagen-supporting foods into your meals:

Day 1

Breakfast: Smoothie of blueberries

Lunch: Spinach salad

Dinner: Steamed broccoli along with grilled chicken breast

Day 2

Breakfast: Berries, sauteed vegetables and eggs

Lunch: Steamed spinach and baked sweet potato

Dinner: Braised beef with thyme and garlic

Day 3

Breakfast: Omelet (include, mushroom, onions, potato, and red bell pepper in the omelet)

Lunch: Quinoa salad that includes basil, honey, berries, chicken breast, and quinoa

Dinner: Turkey meatballs, roasted spaghetti squash and asparagus

Day 4

Breakfast: make a frittata consisting of veggies and eggs

Lunch: Salsa chicken salad

Dinner: Chicken bone broth

Day 5

Breakfast: Banana, Blueberries, and Almond Milk Smoothie

Lunch: Lettuce-wrapped bison burger (tomatoes, smashed avocado, lettuce, cauliflower, and carrots to be added to bison patty)

Dinner: Steamed veggies added to New York strip steak

Day 6

Breakfast: Protein pitaya smoothie (a mixture of pineapple, coconut water, and dragon fruit) plus steamed veggies of your choice

Lunch: Lettuce-wrapped Bison burger

Dinner: Braised beef

Day 7

(any combinations that you felt you enjoyed before this day; it's your choice)

Now that you have an idea of different combinations, it's your turn to be creative considering variety, color, taste, caloric content, and perhaps, budget.

Do include the recipes in the next chapter including the salmon recipes.

Sample Recipes for Collagen Diet

Avocado Deviled Eggs

Ingredients:

- 6 large eggs
- 1 ripe avocado
- 2 tsp. of lime juice (to preserve color and add a zesty flavor)
- 1/4 teaspoon of garlic powder
- Salt and pepper to taste
- A pinch of paprika (for garnish)
- Fresh cilantro (optional, for garnish)
- 1 Tbsp. of olive oil (rich in healthy fats, supporting skin health)

Instructions:

1. Boil the Eggs: Place eggs in a saucepan and cover with water. Bring to a boil, then cover and remove from heat. Let stand for 12 minutes. Afterward, transfer the eggs to a bowl of ice water to cool.
2. Prepare the Avocado Mixture: While the eggs are cooling, peel and pit the avocado. In a bowl, mash the avocado with lime juice, garlic powder, salt, pepper, and olive oil until smooth and creamy. Adjust seasoning to your taste.
3. Peel and Halve the Eggs: Once cooled, peel the eggs and cut them in half lengthwise. Gently remove the

yolks and add them to the avocado mixture. Mix until well combined and smooth.
4. Fill the Egg Whites: Spoon or pipe the avocado and yolk mixture back into the hollows of the egg whites. Be generous, and make sure each egg half is filled.
5. Garnish and Serve: Sprinkle a pinch of paprika over the eggs for a touch of color and flavor. If you like, top each egg half with a small leaf of fresh cilantro for an extra burst of freshness.
6. Chill Before Serving: For the best flavor, chill the prepared avocado-deviled eggs in the refrigerator for about 30 minutes before serving. This allows the flavors to meld together beautifully.

Braised Beef with Garlic and Thyme

Ingredients:

- 2 lbs beef chuck roast (a great source of collagen due to its connective tissues)
- Salt and black pepper to taste
- 2 Tbsp. olive oil
- 8 cloves garlic, minced
- 1 large onion, finely chopped
- 2 carrots, peeled and sliced
- 2 stalks celery, sliced
- 2 cups beef broth (additional source of collagen and hydration)
- 1/2 cup red wine (optional, adds depth; can be replaced with extra beef broth if preferred)
- 4 sprigs fresh thyme (or 1 tsp dried thyme)
- 2 bay leaves

Instructions:

1. Prep the Beef: Season the beef chuck roast generously with salt and black pepper on all sides.
2. Brown the Beef: In a large Dutch oven or heavy-bottomed pot, heat the olive oil over medium-high heat. Add the beef and sear until browned on all sides, about 3-4 minutes per side. Remove the beef from the pot and set aside.

3. Sauté the Vegetables: In the same pot, add the minced garlic, chopped onion, sliced carrots, and celery. Sauté until the vegetables are softened and the onions are translucent for about 5-7 minutes.
4. Deglaze and Add the Beef Back: Pour in the red wine (or extra beef broth) to deglaze the pan, scraping up any browned bits from the bottom of the pot with a wooden spoon. Allow the liquid to reduce by half, then return the beef to the pot.
5. Add Liquids and Herbs: Pour in the beef broth until it just covers the beef. Add the thyme sprigs and bay leaves. Bring the mixture to a simmer.
6. Braise: Cover the pot with a tight-fitting lid and reduce the heat to low. Allow the beef to braise slowly for about 3 hours, or until it is incredibly tender and falls apart easily.
7. Final Touches: Once the beef is tender, remove it from the pot and shred it gently with two forks. If desired, you can reduce the sauce further by simmering it on the stove until it thickens to your liking. Discard the bay leaves and thyme sprigs.
8. Serve: Return the shredded beef to the pot to mix with the sauce and vegetables. Adjust seasoning with additional salt and pepper if necessary. Serve hot, garnished with fresh thyme leaves.

Raw Kale Salad

Ingredients:

- 1 bunch of fresh kale (stems removed and leaves finely chopped)
- 1 avocado, diced
- 1/2 cup of thinly sliced red bell pepper (rich in vitamin C, which aids collagen synthesis)
- one-fourth cup of red onion, thinly sliced
- 1/2 cup of chopped walnuts (omega-3 fatty acids for skin health)
- 1 Tbsp. of sesame seeds (for added texture and minerals)
- one-fourth cup of extra virgin olive oil (healthy fats to support collagen absorption)
- 2 Tbsp. of lemon juice (vitamin C boosts collagen production)
- 1 clove garlic, minced (sulfur supports collagen synthesis)
- Salt and black pepper to taste
- Optional: Add 1 teaspoon of either honey or pure maple syrup to sweeten.

Instructions:

1. Prepare the Kale: Place chopped kale in a large mixing bowl. Add a pinch of salt and massage the kale with your hands for about 2-3 minutes, or until the kale

starts to soften and wilt. This process helps in breaking down the fibrous leaves, making them easier to digest and more palatable.
2. Make the Dressing: In a small bowl, whisk together the extra virgin olive oil, lemon juice, minced garlic, and optional honey or maple syrup. Season with salt and black pepper to taste.
3. Combine the Salad: To the massaged kale, add the diced avocado, sliced red bell pepper, red onion, chopped walnuts, and sesame seeds. Toss gently to combine.
4. Dress the Salad: Pour the dressing over the salad and toss again, ensuring all the ingredients are well coated with the dressing.
5. Serve: Allow the salad to sit for about 10 minutes before serving. This resting time lets the kale absorb the dressing, further softening the leaves and enhancing the flavors.
6. Garnish: Optionally, garnish with additional sesame seeds or a sprinkle of chili flakes for a bit of heat.

Bone Broth

Ingredients:

- 2 pounds of mixed beef bones (knuckles, joints, marrow bones – grass-fed recommended)
- 2 carrots, roughly chopped
- 2 celery stalks, roughly chopped
- 1 onion, quartered (skin on is okay for extra color and nutrients)
- 4 cloves of garlic, smashed
- 2 bay leaves
- A few sprigs of fresh thyme (Alternatively, use 1 teaspoon of dried thyme)
- 1 Tbsp. apple cider vinegar (helps extract minerals and collagen from the bones)
- 12 cups of water (or enough to cover the bones by a couple of inches)
- Salt and pepper to taste

Instructions:

1. Prep the Bones: For a deeper flavor, roast the bones before simmering. Preheat your oven to 400°F (200°C), place the bones on a baking sheet, and roast for 30 minutes.
2. Combine Ingredients: Put roasted bones, carrots, celery, onion, garlic, bay leaves, and thyme into a large stockpot or slow cooker. Add apple cider vinegar and

water to cover the bones completely. Lightly season with salt and pepper.
3. Slow Cook: Bring the mixture to a boil, then reduce the heat to a simmer. For a stockpot, cover partially with a lid and simmer for 12-24 hours; the longer, the better to fully extract the collagen. If using a slow cooker, set it to low and cook for the same duration.
4. Skim the Fat: Throughout the cooking process, skim off any foam or excess fat that rises to the surface with a spoon.
5. Strain the Broth: After simmering, remove from heat and let cool slightly. Strain the broth through a fine-mesh sieve or cheesecloth to remove the solids. Discard the solids.
6. Cool and Store: Allow the broth to cool to room temperature. If desired, refrigerate overnight. Any excess fat will solidify at the top and can be easily removed if preferred.
7. Serve or Store: You can serve the broth warm, season to taste, or use it as a base for soups and stews. For storage, the broth can be kept in the refrigerator for up to 5 days or frozen in small batches for up to 3 months.

Seared Salmon

Ingredients:

- 4 salmon filets (6 ounces each, skin-on, preferably wild-caught for higher omega-3 content)
- 2 Tbsp. olive oil
- Salt and freshly ground black pepper, to taste
- 1 lemon, sliced into rounds
- 2 cloves garlic, minced
- Add 1 teaspoon of thyme leaves, freshly picked (or dried thyme if fresh is unavailable)
- Optional garnish: A sprinkle of chopped parsley or dill for additional flavor and color

Instructions:

1. Prepare the Salmon: Begin by patting the salmon filets dry with paper towels. This step is crucial for achieving a nice sear. Season both sides of the salmon liberally with salt and pepper.
2. Heat the Pan: Heat the olive oil in a large non-stick skillet or frying pan over medium-high heat. The oil should be hot but not smoking.
3. Cook the Salmon: Place the salmon skin-side down in a hot pan. Cook for 4-5 minutes until the skin is crisp. Flip the filets, and add garlic and lemon slices around them. Add thyme on top. Cook for another 3-4 minutes

for medium doneness, until it flakes easily with a fork. Cooking time depends on filet thickness.
4. Garnish and Serve: Once cooked, transfer the salmon filets to plates. You can spoon some of the garlic and lemon-infused oil from the pan over the top for added flavor. Garnish with fresh parsley or dill, if using.
5. Enjoy: Serve the seared salmon immediately, accompanied by a side of steamed vegetables or a fresh salad for a balanced, collagen-friendly meal.

Steamed Salmon

Ingredients:

- 4 salmon filets (about 6 ounces each, skin-on, preferably wild-caught)
- 1 Tbsp. extra virgin olive oil
- Salt and freshly ground black pepper, to taste
- 1 lemon, thinly sliced
- 2 Tbsp. fresh dill, chopped (plus extra for garnish)
- 1 garlic clove, minced
- Optional: Slices of ginger (for added anti-inflammatory benefits)

Instructions:

1. Prepare the Steamer: Fill the bottom of a steamer pot with water, making sure the water level is low enough not to touch the bottom of the steamer basket when it's placed inside. Bring the water to a simmer.
2. Season the Salmon: Brush each salmon filet with extra virgin olive oil. Season with salt and pepper. Top with lemon slices and chopped dill. Optionally, add ginger slices for extra flavor and health benefits.
3. Arrange in Steamer: Line the steamer basket with parchment or cabbage leaves to stop the salmon from sticking. Place the salmon filets in the basket, spaced out for even cooking.

4. Steam the Salmon: Put the steamer basket over simmering water and cover with a tight lid. Steam the salmon for 6-8 minutes or until it's cooked through and easily flakes with a fork. Cooking time varies with filet thickness.
5. Garnish and Serve: Carefully remove the salmon filets from the steamer. Discard the lemon slices and ginger (if used). Garnish the filets with fresh dill and a squeeze of lemon juice before serving.
6. Enjoy: Serve the steamed salmon immediately, with a side of steamed vegetables like asparagus, broccoli, or a mixed greens salad for a complete, collagen-supportive meal.

New York Strip Steak

Ingredients:

- 4 New York strip steaks
- Salt and pepper, to taste
- 1 Tbsp. extra virgin olive oil
- 3 Tbsp. unsalted butter
- 4 cloves garlic, minced
- Optional: Fresh herbs, such as rosemary or thyme (for added flavor)

Instructions:

1. Prepare the Steaks: Let the steaks sit at room temperature for 30 minutes before cooking. Dry them with paper towels to remove excess moisture for a better sear.
2. Season the Steaks: Rub each steak with a tablespoon of extra virgin olive oil, then season both sides with salt and freshly ground black pepper. Press minced garlic onto both sides, using the oil to help it stick.
3. Preheat the Pan: Heat a cast-iron skillet or heavy frying pan over medium-high heat until very hot. No need to add additional oil due to the oil already applied to the steaks.
4. Cook the Steaks: Put the steaks in the hot pan with rosemary and thyme. Cook for 4-5 minutes per side for

medium-rare or adjust for your preferred doneness. Flip the steaks with tongs for even cooking.
5. Rest the Steaks: Once cooked, move the steaks to a cutting board or plate. Cover loosely with aluminum foil and let them rest for 5-10 minutes. Resting is key for juicy, tender, and flavorful steak.
6. Deglaze the Pan (Optional): After removing the steaks, make a simple sauce by reheating the pan. Deglaze with red wine vinegar, scraping up browned bits. Simmer until slightly reduced, then drizzle over the steaks to serve.
7. Serve: After resting, slice the steaks against the grain into thick slices if desired. Serve right away with pan sauce and a side like a fresh green salad or roasted vegetables for a complete, collagen-supportive meal.

Lettuce-Wrapped Bison Burger

Ingredients:

- 1 lb. ground bison meat
- 1 tsp salt
- 1/2 tsp black pepper
- 1 tbsp Worcestershire sauce
- 2 cloves minced garlic
- Lettuce leaves for wrapping burgers (such as iceberg or romaine)

Instructions:

1. Prepare the Bison Patties: In a bowl, mix ground bison, garlic powder, onion powder, salt, and black pepper. Gently combine to avoid tough patties. Shape into 4 equal patties.
2. Cook the Patties: Heat olive oil in a skillet on medium-high. Add bison patties and cook for 3-4 minutes per side, or until done to your liking.
3. Prepare the "Buns": While the patties are cooking, prepare your lettuce leaves. Choose large, sturdy leaves that can hold the burger and toppings. Wash and pat them dry.
4. Assemble the Burgers: Place each cooked bison patty on a lettuce leaf. Top with slices of avocado, tomato, and red onion. If using, add mustard, homemade mayo, or a splash of apple cider vinegar for extra flavor.

5. Wrap and Serve: Carefully fold the lettuce around the contents, tucking in the edges as much as possible to secure the wrap. Serve immediately.

Veggie and Egg Frittata

Ingredients:

- 8 large eggs (preferably organic, free-range for higher nutritional content)
- 1/2 cup full-fat coconut milk (for creaminess and healthy fats)
- Salt and freshly ground black pepper, to taste
- 2 Tbsp. olive oil
- 1 small onion, finely chopped
- 2 cloves garlic, minced
- 1 cup spinach, roughly chopped
- 1/2 cup cherry tomatoes, halved
- 1/2 red bell pepper, diced (rich in vitamin C, aiding in collagen synthesis)
- one-fourth cup fresh basil leaves, chopped (plus more for garnish)
- Optional: one-fourth cup grated Parmesan cheese (if dairy is included in your version of the collagen diet)

Instructions:

1. Preheat the Oven: Preheat your oven to 375°F (190°C), ensuring it's up to temperature before you start baking the frittata.
2. Whisk Eggs and Coconut Milk: In a medium bowl, whisk together the eggs, coconut milk, salt, and pepper until well combined. Set aside.

3. Sauté Veggies: Heat olive oil in a skillet (like cast iron) over medium heat. Sauté onion and garlic until soft, about 2-3 minutes. Add spinach, cherry tomatoes, and red bell pepper, and cook until spinach wilts and veggies soften, about 3-5 minutes.
4. Combine Eggs with Veggies: Pour the egg mix into the skillet with sautéed veggies. Stir to distribute eggs evenly. Top with basil and Parmesan (if used).
5. Bake the Frittata: Move the skillet to the oven. Bake for 20-25 minutes, until the eggs set and the top turns golden. A knife inserted in the center should come out clean.
6. Garnish and Serve: Once done, remove from the oven and let it cool for a few minutes. Garnish with additional fresh basil before slicing into wedges and serving.

Spinach Salad

Ingredients:

- 1 cup spinach leaves, washed and dried
- 1/2 avocado, diced (contains vitamin E, an antioxidant that helps protect collagen)
- one-fourth cup chopped almonds or walnuts (rich in omega-3 fatty acids, which help maintain skin elasticity)
- one-fourth cup of crumbled feta cheese (if dairy is included in your version of the collagen diet)

Instructions:

1. Prepare the Dressing: In a small bowl, whisk together the extra virgin olive oil, apple cider vinegar, honey (if using), salt, and pepper until well combined. Adjust the seasoning to your taste.
2. Assemble the Salad: In a large salad bowl, mix spinach leaves, sliced strawberries, blueberries, and chopped walnuts. Gently toss to combine.
3. Add Avocado and Optional Cheese: Add the sliced avocado to the salad, and if you're including cheese, sprinkle the crumbled feta or goat cheese over the top.
4. Dress the Salad: Drizzle the prepared dressing over the salad just before serving. Gently toss everything together to ensure the salad is evenly coated with the dressing.

5. Garnish and Serve: If using, garnish the salad with chia or flax seeds for extra nutrients. Serve immediately for a fresh, flavorful addition to your collagen diet.

Turkey Meatballs

Ingredients:

- 1 lb ground turkey (look for lean, organic if possible)
- one-fourth cup almond flour (as a healthier, grain-free breadcrumb alternative)
- 1 large egg (helps with binding and is also good for collagen production)
- one-fourth cup finely chopped fresh parsley
- 2 cloves garlic, minced
- 1 teaspoon onion powder
- 1/2 tsp. sea salt
- 1/4 tsp. black pepper
- 1 Tbsp. olive oil (for cooking)
- Optional: 1 Tbsp. collagen powder (to boost the collagen content)

Instructions:

1. Prep Work: In a large mixing bowl, combine the ground turkey, almond flour, egg, chopped parsley, minced garlic, onion powder, sea salt, black pepper, and optional collagen powder. Mix well until all ingredients are evenly distributed.
2. Form Meatballs: Once your mixture is ready, start forming it into meatballs. Depending on your preference, you can make them bite-sized or slightly

larger. Usually, this mixture yields around 15-20 meatballs.

3. Cooking: Heat the olive oil in a large skillet over medium heat. Once the oil is hot, add the meatballs. Cook them for about 7-10 minutes, turning occasionally, until they're golden brown on all sides and cooked through. The internal temperature should reach at least 165°F (74°C) when checked with a meat thermometer.

4. Serving Suggestion: Serve these delicious turkey meatballs over a bed of fresh greens, zucchini noodles, or steamed vegetables like broccoli or cauliflower. These sides are not only complementary to the meatballs but are also excellent for a collagen-boosting diet.

5. Optional: For an added touch, you can whip up a quick sauce by blending roasted red peppers, olive oil, garlic, and a touch of vinegar. This sauce pairs wonderfully with the meatballs and keeps the dish within the guidelines of the collagen diet.

Conclusion

Thank you deeply for joining us on this enlightening voyage through the ins and outs of the collagen diet. By reaching this point, you've armed yourself with invaluable knowledge about one of the most fundamental proteins in our bodies. You've ventured beyond the surface, uncovering how integrating collagen into your diet can significantly enhance your health, from revitalizing skin to fortifying bones and joints.

Collagen's role in our wellness cannot be overstated. It acts as the glue that holds us together, and by prioritizing its place in our diets, you're setting the stage for a healthier, more vibrant version of yourself. The insights shared in this guide are more than just pathways to improved physical appearance; they are stepping stones towards a lifestyle enriched with well-being and vitality.

Now, equipped with a deeper understanding of collagen's benefits, you understand that incorporating it into your diet goes beyond mere aesthetic improvements. You've learned that it plays a critical role in supporting joint health, enhancing gut function, and promoting heart health, among other benefits. This knowledge empowers you to make informed choices about your nutrition, choices that ripple out to affect all areas of your health.

The beauty of the collagen diet lies in its simplicity and flexibility. Whether through natural food sources like bone broth, leafy greens, berries, and garlic or through supplements, you've seen how effortlessly collagen can be woven into the fabric of your daily eating habits. This adaptability ensures that boosting your collagen intake is not just a fleeting trend but a sustainable practice that fits seamlessly into your lifestyle.

Remember, the journey toward optimal health is a personal one. Each step you take, each choice you make, brings you closer to realizing the full potential of your well-being. Be patient and kind to yourself as you adapt to this collagen-rich approach to eating. It's okay to experiment, to find what works best for you and your unique body. After all, true health is about finding balance and harmony within our lives.

We hope this guide has served as a valuable resource, illuminating the path toward integrating collagen into your diet and, by extension, into a holistic approach to your health. May the steps you take from here forward be guided by the insights and knowledge you've gained.

In closing, we extend our sincerest gratitude for allowing us to accompany you on this part of your health and wellness journey. Your dedication to learning about and implementing the collagen diet is commendable, and we're excited about the positive changes that lie ahead for you. Keep pushing forward, stay curious, and continue to nurture your body with the nourishment it deserves.

Here's to a future where every meal brings you closer to your health goals, powered by the strength and resilience that collagen brings to our bodies. Keep striving, keep thriving, and remember—the best investment you will ever make is in your health.

FAQ

What exactly is the collagen diet?

The collagen diet is a nutritional plan focused on increasing your intake of collagen, a protein crucial for skin elasticity, joint health, and overall bodily function. This diet emphasizes consuming collagen-rich foods like bone broth, fish, berries, and leafy greens, as well as taking collagen supplements to support your body's natural collagen production.

How does the collagen diet benefit my skin?

Collagen plays a vital role in maintaining skin's elasticity and hydration. By following a collagen diet, you may see improvements in skin texture and firmness, a reduction in wrinkles, and an overall more youthful appearance due to the diet's focus on collagen-rich foods and supplements that support skin health.

Can the collagen diet help with joint pain?

Yes, the collagen diet can help with joint pain. Collagen supports joint health by maintaining the integrity of cartilage, the rubber-like tissue that protects your joints. An increased intake of collagen has been linked to reduced inflammation and pain in the joints and may improve symptoms of arthritis.

Are there vegetarian or vegan options for the collagen diet?

While collagen is primarily found in animal products, vegetarians and vegans can follow a modified collagen diet by focusing on plant-based foods that promote collagen production. Nutrients like vitamin C, proline, and glycine - found in citrus fruits, soy, black beans, and seeds - are essential for collagen synthesis in the body.

How long does it take to see results from the collagen diet?

Results can vary based on individual health factors and the consistency of following the diet. Generally, people begin to notice changes in skin appearance and joint flexibility within 3 to 6 months of consistently incorporating collagen-rich foods and supplements into their diet.

Are there any side effects of the collagen diet?

The collagen diet is generally safe for most people. However, some individuals may experience mild digestive issues when beginning collagen supplements. It's important to start with lower doses and gradually increase to the recommended dosage to minimize potential side effects. Always consult with a healthcare professional before starting any new dietary plan, especially if you have existing health conditions.

How do I ensure I'm getting enough collagen from my diet?

To ensure you're getting enough collagen from your diet, include a variety of collagen-rich foods such as bone broth, chicken skin, fish, egg whites, and dairy products. Additionally, consider supplementing with a high-quality collagen supplement. Paying attention to other nutrients that support collagen production, like vitamin C and zinc, will further enhance your body's ability to produce and utilize collagen effectively.

References and Helpful Links

Meakin, C., & Meakin, C. (2020, October 21). 8 Collagen benefits: when to take, dosage, supplements, collagen foods and more. Bluebird Provisions. https://bluebirdprovisions.co/blogs/news/benefits-collagen

Bolke, L., Schlippe, G., Gerß, J., & Voss, W. (2019). A collagen supplement improves skin hydration, elasticity, roughness, and density: results of a randomized, Placebo-Controlled, blind study. Nutrients, 11(10), 2494. https://doi.org/10.3390/nu11102494

Collagen in pregnancy: Is it safe? (n.d.). Mother & Baby. https://www.motherandbaby.com/pregnancy/labour-birth/collagen-in-pregnancy/

Cellulite - Symptoms and causes - Mayo Clinic. (2023, November 21). Mayo Clinic. https://www.mayoclinic.org/diseases-conditions/cellulite/symptoms-causes/syc-20354945

Further Food. (n.d.). Further food collagen products and health supplements. https://www.furtherfood.com/

Wu, M., Cronin, K., & Crane, J. S. (2023, September 4). Biochemistry, collagen synthesis. StatPearls - NCBI Bookshelf. https://www.ncbi.nlm.nih.gov/books/NBK507709/

Further Food. (2023, October 11). Why Collagen is a Supplement all Diabetics Should Be Taking. https://www.furtherfood.com/blogs/articles/collagen-protein-stabilize-blood-sugar-diabetes-restore-collagen-production-diabetics

Eucerin. (n.d.). EUCERIN-AS-Male-and-Female-skin-00header. https://int.eucerin.com/about-skin/basic-skin-knowledge/male-and-female-skin#:~:text=Both%20their%20sebaceous%20glands%20and,dry%20skin%20than%20adult%20females.

Professional, C. C. M. (n.d.-b). Collagen. Cleveland Clinic. https://my.clevelandclinic.org/health/articles/23089-collagen

Wu, M., Cronin, K., & Crane, J. S. (2023b, September 4). Biochemistry, collagen synthesis. StatPearls - NCBI Bookshelf. https://www.ncbi.nlm.nih.gov/books/NBK507709/

Van De Walle Ms Rd, G. (2024, January 29). What you need to know about the health benefits of collagen. Healthline. https://www.healthline.com/nutrition/collagen-benefits

www.ingramcontent.com/pod-product-compliance
Lightning Source LLC
LaVergne TN
LVHW012035060526
838201LV00061B/4614